Bernhard J. Schmidt

Plaintext compact

Is my child autistic?

Encouraging answers
to a scary question.

Bernhard J. Schmidt

Plaintext compact
Is my child autistic?
Encouraging answers
to a scary question.

ISBN: 978-3750419742

translated from
Klartext kompakt
Ist (m)ein Kind Autist?
*Ermutigende Antworten auf
eine beängstigende Frage.*
© 2018 Bernhard J. Schmidt
ISBN: 978-3748147503

Production and Publishing:
BoD – Books on Demand, Norderstedt, Germany

Bibliographic information of the German National Library:
The German National Library lists this publication
in the German National Bibliography; detailed bibliographic
Data are available online at http://dnb.dnb.de.

Table of content

I. PREFACE

It is the experience of one year "Solidar Hotel Goldener Stern" with the offer "Holidays for families with (autistic) children", which led me to write this book.

Already in the first year several hundred children were our guests, of which about 50 children, adolescents and adults with an autism diagnosis.

Among the other children, however, were some who showed clear signs of autism - and in which some parents had a "suspicion", others not.

The "abnormalities" of the children were so small that they would not be enough for a diagnosis, but still so that the parents have at least partially considered possible causes.

Be it a delayed language development, little interest in other people or children, problems with motor skills, emotion regulation ...

I would have liked to have told many parents that, in my opinion, their child is an autistic person and therefore they should take this into consideration as the child develops. And also educators, for example, in kindergarten and daycare, are increasingly faced with the question of whether one of the children may be autistic. How to recognize this and what to consider then?

7

The past few decades, however, have given a false picture of autism - of autism as a disease.
A disease that was also presented as an unalterable, non-treatable fate and unfortunately is still. That's why parents alone fear the word "autism" as threatening and frightening.

But autism is not a disease!
Even autistic people can develop normally and lead a happy life as part of society!
These are historical events that have led to the discovery of only the autistic individuals who have experienced massive disruption of development.
Yes, the more bizarre the disorder is, the greater the media interest. "Normal" autistic people just are not spectacular enough to talk about.
What was once the rarities cabinet with two-headed calves, the lady without abdomen, etc. at the fair, these are today the reports of autistics, suffering from a disruption of their development.
The fact that these disturbances can be avoided as a rule, and if they have occurred can then be treated, was and is overlooked.
Autism is a "vulnerability", that is, a vulnerability that causes autism to be more likely to disrupt development - but not necessarily.

As with a red-blond child, the risk of sunburn is greater. However, suitable protective measures can prevent sunburn and, in the case of autistics, a disruption of development.

Therefore it is necessary to educate the parents, but also educators about

1. what is autism,
2. how autism manifests, so that one can recognize the child as autistic,
3. and how to reduce the risk of developing disorders.

Basically, our technological prosperity and achievement society is a permanent overstrain for ALL children. And not only for these. Adults also increasingly suffer from mental disorders.

The increased susceptibility to disruption of development lies only in the lower limit of autism overload.

But that also means that everything that is good for autistic children is good for all other children as well!

So that what promotes the development of autistic children, also promotes all other children.

A false-positive "diagnosis", that is, if one wrongly considers a child to be an autistic, has no harmful consequences - as long as one understands autism correctly. Problems can arise if one ignores the specifics of the child.

This book is not only intended to convey a new understanding, but also to raise awareness of the special developments of autistic people and possible problems.

II. FOUR STORIES AS AN INTRODUCTION

The last 70 years, beginning with the descriptions of autistic patients by Asperger and Kanner, were solely characterized by a purely descriptive (phenomenological-descriptive) "understanding" of autism as a disease. In the last few years, the descriptions of the "professionals" from science and research were supplemented by the "inner views" of autistic people and self-advocacy organizations. However, this has changed nothing about the errors about autism. On the contrary, prejudices were further cemented by this.

I would like to contrast the purely static descriptions that focus on the deficits and those postulated as "God given" by four other perspectives that show the advantages as well as the evolutionary significance of autism.

1   Thalina, the huntress

Dusk was already breaking as Thalina brushed through the forest. The other members of her clan were already in the camp, busy firing the fire. But Thalina did not fear like the others the night and darkness - on the contrary. She was the best hunter in the group and therefore enjoyed great reputation. Because she not only knew all the animals of the forest, but also their behavior, sounds and signals, traces and feces. And she almost always brought rich prey from her forays into the camp.

She lived at a time when humans were not only hunters, but always prey at the same time.

But her hearing and smell were so good that she not only perceived a threat but also prey in time. And her eyes were as sharp as those of an eagle. She also felt neither pain nor cold. While the others sat by the warming campfire and told stories, Thalina roamed the woods, enjoying the altered perception of dusk and darkness. Everything became calm and the smell of the forest was different, moister, more intense. She was better at bow and arrow and spear than others in the clan, climbing trees better than others, which was often useful. Only the fairytale lessons by the fire together with the others - she avoided them. Rather, she explored the area and discovered so many new campsites, sources ...

2   Ben, the alpine dairyman

The sky was still blue, not a cloud in the sky, but Ben was already smelling the rising storm. He tentatively secured the hut and called the animals into the stable. He had been in the mountains for three months, mostly alone with his animals. Radio, mobile phone and tourism were not invented at the time. And no electricity. From time to time a child of the farmer or his wife came to see to it and brought the cheese down to the valley. But most of the time he was alone. He knew all his animals, knew all the plants and all the dangers for himself and his animals, their diseases and also the medicinal herbs that helped. He got up with the sun, and went to bed with the dusk. In between, he worked the whole day, chopping down trees and chopping wood, milking the cows, making cheese ... he did not have much time for himself. There was also no weekend for him - the animals wanted to be taken care of every day. The farmer was very happy with his Ben, because not only did he make good cheese, but he also brought the animals back to the valley in the fall, all healthy. The fact that you could not talk much to Ben about the happenings in the village, was not so important.

3   Sali, the gatherer

There were not many mushrooms in the baskets of the others - Sali saw this already in the distance. His basket was full. For the others, he would also have to sort out some of the few mushrooms that are not edible. He knew all the mushrooms, knew which are eatable and which are not. He knew when and where the best mushrooms were growing - and saw mushrooms that many others had missed without seeing them.

"You look different somehow," the others had once told him.

But he also knew about berries and roots, sat early with the ancients or accompanied them into the forest while the other children played together. So he had learned as a child, what many others could not as adults. You could not talk much to him. But the small-talk, which was not invented at the time, would hardly have had time anyway. And once, when he talked about mushrooms and berries, he did not speak like the others, even though he had grown up among them.

When it was celebrated, it was done according to set rules. But he usually stayed away from it. He preferred to be a soliloquy.

4   Dayal, the monk

It was hot and stuffy in the village, the sun burned down and dazzled. It stank everywhere of sweat, garbage, and decay, and the noise, the chatter, and the running around of the many people, running back and forth like ants, were unbearable. So Dayal rejoiced when he could step through the gates of the monastery - to the peace, the shade, the coolness. Already as a small child his parents had given him to the monastery - at that time he had been somehow different from his many siblings. He preferred to remain alone, looking at flowers and beetles, and kept away from the children's games and struggles.

In the monastery, he enjoyed the clear day structure of prayers, meals and tasks. He loved the solid rituals together with the other monks with whom he had little to do otherwise. He loved the silence.

In the monastery he was considered wise. He spoke little, but what he said was not only appreciated by the other monks.

5 Childhood

All four personalities described, though perhaps hundreds of years between them, grew up in societies and groups that were manageable. In which the group or the village was the "Kita". At a time when most of the day was filled with work and the children had to help as well from an early age. At a time when the children were not yet separated from the work of their parents - and despite all the hard work and hardship there was no burn-out.

Too easy to forget that the televisions are only about 50 years ago moved into the living room, the Internet has only existed for about 20 years ... and smartphones only a few years. Also, the rural exodus and the strong expansion of the cities, the increase in car and air traffic is not so old.

All this has made life more comfortable on the one hand and more stressful on the other.

The greatest need these days is the abundance - also the abundance of perceptual stimuli. In a few epochs of humanity, life has changed as fast and as extensively as in the last 100 years. And so it is not surprising that the first descriptions of autism also emerged only about 70 years ago. Then, forgotten for a few decades, they were rediscovered as the blessings of industrialization were poured out over us to their fullest extent.

As forests became "parks with trim trails" and meadows and pastures became production areas ...

6   Similarities

All protagonists of the four stories have in common that they show clear signs of autism - and all would not be perceived as ill.

These signs of autism, also described in the past, include:

- Hypersensitivity, that is an increased perception by the senses.

- Special form of pattern recognition.

- Good eye-hand coordination.

- Independence from (unconscious) group communication, more loners.

- Strong interest in factual topics and pronounced exploratory behavior.

- Hardly any language, and if so, then relevant.

- By contrast, little interest in fairy tales, small talk ...

- High level of activity, that is a certain amount of restlessness.

- Other pain and temperature perception, as a rule, pain and cold are barely noticed.

- Little to no fear.

And it should also be clear that, depending on the cultural environment, autism may be more beneficial - even for the other people (the group).
Some readers will now also think that the descriptions fit

but quite well on one or the other acquaintances, who lives his life quite normal, with job, partner and children.

III. WHAT IS COMMON TO ALL CHILDREN

The knowledge about the necessary development and learning processes in children seems to have been largely lost. More and more children are being treated like little adults. It is discussed with them as if the cognitive functions were already fully developed, for example in the case of 2-year-olds. The children are confronted with the choice of alternatives, which they often can not overlook due to the still outstanding learning processes. Also, the children are increasingly demanded beyond their load limit. And stress has already entered the nursery today. There are hardly any opportunities for children to retreat between school, violin and ballet.

1 Learning processes

Of course, many of the foundations of our development are already present in us at birth. But many things need to be learned based on these assets. These learning processes involve much more skills than you might think. On the other hand, the learning processes depend on the socio-cultural environment in which they take place. This way, every child is optimally adapted to the respective environment. And all these learning processes require a lot of energy - and therefore also rest and relaxation for the learners.

Children also learn a lot by playing together. One of the biggest mistakes in autism is that autistic children do not want to and can not play with other children. But also autistic children want and can play. It's just harder for them. For example, if one child withdraws from the others in kindergarten and sorts the cars by size, then that is neither a sign for not wanting nor for being not able to play. As a rule, however, the child is overwhelmed with the overall situation and therefore withdraws into his own world.

1.1   Regulation of bodily functions

Both the sleep / wake cycle, digestion and cleanliness are also learned through environmental orientation based on the maturation of bodily functions.

But also the senses like seeing, hearing, smelling, feeling are adapted by the interaction with the environment - this is called "sensory integration". The child learns to classify and understand the perceptions. Thus the world, which we always perceive through at least one of the senses, becomes understandable for the children.

1.2 Regulation of Aggression, Exploration and Emotions

Also innate are aggression and exploration as behaviors necessary for survival. In a less well-organized affluent society like ours, aggression and exploration were still needed to find and defend habitats, food, and sexual partners. However, the handling of these behaviors has to be learned. This, too, can be very different, depending on the culture. In some cultures, for example, aggression is more accepted, in others less.

And also the evaluation of events, ie which emotions "fit" to an event and to what extent this emotion is to be shown, all this depends on and is learned in this socio-cultural environment.

1.3 Social interaction

Of course, the ability to socialize is also innate. However, the rules and behaviors of each group and culture must be learned by participating in it, for example by playing together.

1.3.a   Language

The ability to communicate through language is a central feature of human beings. Thus, learning the respective language is an essential part of the development of children. Because above all, they can participate in social interaction through language.

Language has, and this is mostly overlooked, much less the function of factual information exchange, so for example to inform other people about the latest bargain at the discount store (formerly, a few hundred years ago, it would have been new food sources).

Speech primarily serves the unconscious communication of belonging to the in-group, namely by imitation of the speech melody of the counterpart, adoption of dialects and phrases ...

And thus at the same time to the demarcation of foreign groups: "Who does not speak like us, who does not belong to us."

Irony and humor, too, are learned through participation in social interaction within a socio-cultural environment.

Not without reason, for example, we partly have our dear need with the humor in other countries.

Behaviors such as looking in the eyes, giving the hand, showing emotions, are culturally different and are learned through participation in the culture, including through social interaction.

2 Interaction skills

Through the previously described learning processes, the child develops "interaction competence", that is, that he understands his physical (the world of the senses) as well as social (the world of interaction with other living beings) environment, and with this world and other living beings, especially people, can interact.
And that the child finds his way in his socio-cultural world, so that he can orient himself without outside help. The following chapters are intended to sensitize parents and educators for the different developmental areas and to contribute to a better understanding of the stage of development of the child.

3 Requirements

The necessary learning processes that lead to interaction competence have some prerequisites for a successful course.

3.1   Energy - after tired comes stupid

Life in itself is the constant struggle against entropy
under the expense of energy. That without appropriate
energy supply, there is no life.
Learning processes, especially in toddlers and children,
require a lot of additional energy.
And maintaining the regulatory mechanisms that control
aggression, for example, also requires energy. If it lacks
the necessary energy, the regulatory mechanisms
collapse.
"After tired comes stupid" summarizes this in apt words.
For autists, this is called "melt down" - sounds a bit better
- but is the same.

3.2   Orientation

Until their own structures and orientation skills are
developed, the children need external guidance. Through
these children could find their way even in an increasingly complex world. Unfortunately, these external
guidelines are becoming more and more lost.
The dissolution of rigid social structures and behaviors
means additional opportunities for adults to develop, but

it becomes more difficult for children to get their bearings.

For example, the shift work of the parents complicates the development of the sleep / wake cycle.

But the limits of social action are also inquired about by children through the combination of exploration and aggression. Frequently, the children no longer receive clear answers to the question of where the boundaries are. The natural orientation of the children to the parents often revolves, and the parents are based instead on their child. But children are completely overwhelmed with the role of the "leader".

3.3   Relaxation

Fear and stress stand in the way of participation in social interaction. Through fear and stress, the person gets into a "fight or flight" state, which is not suitable for social interaction. Autism has so far been equated with the "flight" state, ie the retreat into its own understandable world of rituals and stereotypes, the sorting of cars instead of playing with them.

The "fight" type has been overlooked so far. So children who do not retreat in response to anxiety and stress, but who are very keen to explore their environment, including threats, and who are more prone to aggression

towards others than to auto-aggression.
But anxiety and stress are always the causes of these children's behavior, whether it's flight or fight.
Therefore relaxation and tranquility would be especially important for children. Only in this condition can they successfully participate in the environment, play together and thus develop in a socio-cultural environment.
Stress is also generated by sensory influences such as noise etc. So nowadays children are often under constant stress. If not by noise, light pollution ... then by a series of activities and tasks. Everything planned for the well-being and development of the child by well-intentioned parents. But the necessary rest and informality often comes too short.

3.4   Participation in social interaction

Unfortunately, participation in social interaction in our society is no longer self-evident.
Even if the children want, and have the necessary energy and peace, they are increasingly excluded from social interaction. For example, through child poverty or disability.
Those who are not like the others, who deviate from the norm, are often excluded from participating in social interaction.

IV. WHAT IS DIFFERENT ABOUT AUTISTIC PEOPLE?

The emphasis is on, and you can not repeat that often enough, on DIFFERENT! So it's not about "sick", "disabled" ... but about another form of perception and behavior that, as shown in the stories, is quite legitimate. But how are autistic people different?

1   Orientation

At the time of Leo Kanner and Hans Asperger, who both independently described autistic children, social psychology was still in its infancy. The findings about the coexistence of people, conscious and unconscious, was not available at the time.

Thus, both Kanner and Asperger described the conspicuous behavior of autistic children without, however, having an explanation for it.

Ultimately, 70 years later, you're not one step further, but you've been spinning in circles so far.

Although hundreds and thousands of "cases" and peculiarities have been described, as well as that autistics show little to no facial expressions, do not imitate the other person, often have a monotonous or no language, do not understand the meaning of small-talk and hardly participate in it ... that autistics often have difficulties with irony and phrases. However, over the years it has not been possible to combine all of these descriptions into one unified theory.

1.1 Social Psychological Perspectives

The results of social psychology, however, not only explain what autism is, but also how, as a consequence of a disruption of social interaction, this can lead to a disruption of development.

1.2 Autism as a lack of unconscious group communication

Exactly about the behaviors that autistics do not show, namely facial expressions, imitation, synchronization, etc. NT people (neurotypical people - not autistic) unconsciously communicate with each other.
Above all, this communication serves to define and maintain one's own group.
By imitating the others, the behavior of the group is also taken over. For example, language and dialects, movement patterns, and speech patterns are learned as

part of the group definition by participating in the group's social interaction.

This unconscious group communication and interaction also serves NT children and adults as an "autopilot", that is, as an automatic orientation.

This is especially helpful when external orientation options are missing.

Autists lack this "autopilot" because they do not participate in the unconscious group communication.

Autistic people always have to be aware and active - and this is particularly difficult in new, unknown situations, such as the first visit to a kindergarten or nursery school, and without external orientation.

2   Energy

In humans, there are two distinct, separate patterns of activity. First, the "task mode", in which, as the name implies, tasks and challenges are solved. Everyone has this. On the other hand, NT people still have a "Relaxation" or "Normal Mode" that comes into action when there are no problems or tasks to solve. This "normal mode" also includes the unconscious group communication, ie small-talk, imitation, synchronization ... so the "autopilot", which also acts as an energy-saving mode. Autists, on the other hand, are always in "task mode". This is why autistic people often show a strong interest in the environment, technical problems, pronounced exploratory behavior ...

Autists do not imitate other people and do not synchronize with them. Imitation, for example, teaches motor movement patterns. This is why autistic people often have problems with motor development.

But above all, the "autopilot" as energy-saving mode is missing. All activities of Autists take place in the "Task Mode" and thus consume a lot of energy, which makes autistic children run out of energy.

In a technical and overstimulated environment, the challenges of hypersensitivity and irritant filter weakness in autistic individuals are added.

The automatic filtering out of disturbing noises (stimulus filter), does not work, but must be operated actively and at the expense of energy. And even with the necessary energy filtering out does not always succeed. The ticking of the clock then has the same meaning and intensity of the perception as the voice of the counterpart.

3 Relaxation

For autistic people and their families, there are very high stress levels. In the case of autistic individuals, these arise due to the sensory peculiarities, but also because of the lack of unconscious group communication. The behaviors of other people often appear to autistics as incomprehensible and puzzling.

Without "normal mode", autistics are also in a permanent "task mode", often without being able to live it out as necessary.

Relaxation as the basis for communication and interaction is therefore a major problem for autistics.

As a rule, fear and stress dominate the lives of autistic people. And these are opposed to social interaction and thus to development.

Here, rest and retreat options can be helpful, as well as changing games that are not only aimed at the (unconscious) imitation, etc., but include the joint problem solving.

V. CONSEQUENCES

Due to the massive, cultural changes in the environment formerly quite positive characteristics can become problems. Autistic people find it more difficult to orient themselves. And this is especially noticeable in an environment where many outward orientations have been lost.

Thus, the world has become more incomprehensible to autistics, often resulting in a retreat from social (as opposed to unconscious) group communication, or challenging behavior.

The world out there is scary.

By shifting from the "task" mode, which shaped society a hundred years ago, into "normal" mode or "small-talk" mode in a prosperous society, more emphasis is placed on unconscious group communication. People who do not show it, including autistic people, are marginalized and often victims of bullying.

This is rare in the kindergarten, because the group perception (I am part of the own group in contrast to the foreign group) in children in kindergarten age is not yet developed.

But at the latest from the transition to school then this will be a problem.

Due to the lack of the "autopilot", especially the imitation, all learning processes can last longer, especially the development of interaction skills. These difficulties increase the risk for autistic individuals that "disturbance of social interaction", and subsequently, a profound "disruption of development" occurs.

1   Risks / vulnerability

By a
1.   sensory and / or
2.   social

(long-term) exposure beyond the exposure limit, which is lower in autistic people than in NT people, and the concomitant permanently high levels of stress, it can lead to the development of physical and mental illness.
But even that does not have to happen if the child's signals, for example that the energy is exhausted or the environment is too loud at the moment, are taken into account.
To avoid the development of disturbances, it is therefore necessary to maintain a load balance. This does not mean that the autistic children can not be burdened beyond the limit of exposure - but this should not be done as a permanent condition.

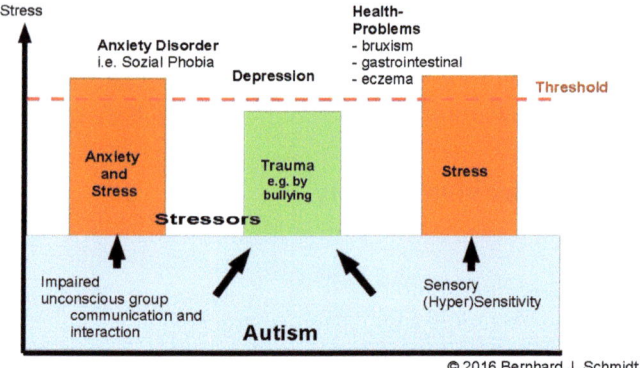

By

1. exclusion or withdrawal of social interaction,
2. lack of external orientation, as well
3. longer learning processes

there is a risk of insufficient development of interaction skills. If then the next higher level of interaction competence is required, for example by attending a kindergarten or enrollment, without the necessary competences being developed, the regression or dissociation of development can occur depending on the age.

Regression mainly occurs in the transition area from toddler to child. Autistic children, who have already spoken and were clean, for example, lose their language and wet themselves up again as a result of the high demands placed on their interaction skills. This repeatedly occurs in autistic children entering the kindergarten or in the day care center.

If the excessive demand or even a bullying / violence experience occurs during the transition from child to adolescent, the result may be a dissociation of development, that is, a separation of development. Although cognitive development then proceeds normally, the socio-emotional development remains at the child's level.

Sensitive phases of development

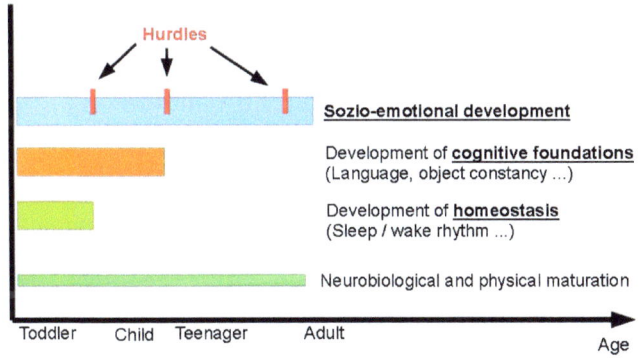

© 2016 Bernhard J. Schmidt

VI. PREVENTION

Even autistic children can develop normally!
Even autistic children can and want to play together with other children!
The risks mentioned above are just risks and not an unalterable fate. It is therefore important to increase sensitivity and anticipatory prevention so that there is no disturbance of social interaction and, as a consequence, disruption of development. And this prevention benefits all children, whether autistic or not.
The answer to the question "Is my child autistic?" serves only to clarify how strongly this prevention should be pronounced. For autistic children may take longer to develop and are more prone to disorders.

1   Pay attention to the load balance

If you decide to go to a gym, you will not start by choosing the maximum exercise load at the beginning. Slowly you will start and slowly increase the loads. With each workout your load limit will increase a little. They will avoid overloading, as they carry the risk of injury. Also, you will not train every day and not many hours, but allow your body time for rest. Only then can the training have a positive effect.

It is similar in both sensory and social development.
These need time and training. However, a burden above
the load limit carries the risk of "injury".

And even a permanent load does not promote the
development, but rather harms it.

However, our society is overburdened by sensory
overload. And this often beyond the limits of stress. This
means that the corresponding stimulus is perceived as
painful and / or threatening. Thus, the body gets into a
prolonged state of stress. And stress, as we have seen,
hinders social interaction. If a child withdraws in
kindergarten or develops challenging behavior, then this
may be the cause.

But also the social interaction skills have to be
developed.

Social interaction is learned through social interaction.
This development also happens through levels of
competency, meaning that the child is not from the
beginning in a position to enter into social interaction
with everyone. First, the ability is limited to one-to-one
communication with parents and family, then to group
communication with friends and acquaintances of the
family, then with strangers.

Many parents experience how difficult the transition from
one communication level to another can be when their

child first visits a kindergarten, for example. The child is required to find herself without the parents in a new environment with strangers; that's a big challenge.
In autistic children, the risk is particularly high that this change comes to problems because the necessary interaction skills have not yet been developed.

2 Attention to the development of interaction skills

If the next level is required on the ladder of interaction by the child, then the child must also have the necessary skills. Autistic children also develop these skills - but sometimes they take longer. Therefore, especially in autistic children a special sensitivity to completed or pending developmental steps is necessary.
Interaction skills include:
1. sensory integration
2. Orientability
3. cognitive development
4. socio-emotional development
5. Communication competence

2.1   Sensory Integration

As already mentioned, in autistic children sensory hypersensitivity often occurs and a stimulus filter weakness is observed. These can stand in the way of sensory integration. But only when the sensory stimuli of the environment can be perceived as understandable and normal, the child can interact meaningfully with the environment.

2.2   Orientation

Can the child orientate in the environment? This is learned on the one hand by external orientation aids such as clear structures and processes, on the other hand also by unconscious group orientation. Since the latter is missing in autistic children, the outer orientation aids are particularly important in the beginning.
But as a target, autistic children should be able to orient themselves in this world, even in new, unknown environments. Even autistic children can learn this. Necessary for the development of the orientation are thereby also the pointing out of (social) borders, furthermore above all also praise, which is often forgotten, and censure, as well as the "measure

regulation" of exploratory behavior and aggression. Without imitation of the behavior of the group and without "autopilot", autistic children understandably need much more external guidance to support the learning process - but often they do not get enough or too little.

2.3   Cognitive development

For the children covered in this book, who only have initial suspicions due to delays in development, one can expect a normal development of cognitive abilities. In our rationalistic world, cognitive development is also overrated, which is why it has largely been overlooked that autistic children have problems with socio-emotional development. However, promotion of these should come first. And this requires social interaction, be it in kindergarten or at school. The emerging online schools, on the other hand, follow the wrong path of pure cognitive development.

2.4   Socio-emotional development

The whole range and complexity of the socio-emotional development comes into focus above all through the analysis of the problems of autistic children. Developments that are usually automatic thanks to "autopilot" and imitation require more effort and energy from autistic children. But even with many neuro-typical children, there are increasing problems in the socio-emotional development.

2.4.a   Frustration tolerance

Nowadays, satisfaction is within reach for every need. For example, there are almost everywhere the big billboards of the burger-roasters, which both arouse and satisfy needs. Hardly the children learn that not every desire and every need is immediately satisfied.
Often the parents fulfill wishes in anticipatory obedience, which the child had not yet uttered.
This way the children hardly experience any frustration - and do not learn to handle it. Even short waiting times when eating or the like then lead to dramas.

2.4.b   Impulse control

Adults too have many impulses, including aggressive as well as peaceful ones. But adults do not usually go after them. On the other hand, anyone who pursues his aggressive impulses uncontrollably, as is increasingly reported in the media, ends up in court.
Children must first learn to deal with and control their

impulses. This learning process also requires social interaction and the identification of social boundaries.

2.4.c   Attention span

In order to get in contact with other people as well as the environment, a developed attention span is needed. If this is insufficiently developed and takes only seconds or minutes, a meaningful interaction is hardly possible. This attention span should not only refer to stereotypical patterns of action with a few objects, but to a flexible interaction with different people and objects.
Often, too high anxiety and stress levels prevent a longer attention span. The children are then in a permanent "fight or flight mode", which makes them restless.

2.4.d   Emotion regulation

Not only the expression and assignment of emotions to events is learned socially, also the regulation of one's own emotions has to be learned. On the one hand, this requires the necessary energy to regulate the emotions. On the other hand, the development of self-esteem. This does not arise in isolation in the child, but through social processes, ie ultimately through participation in social groups.

Success stories and positive feedback are important for all children. The peculiarities of the possible behavior of autistics should not deter this.

2.5   Communication competence

Even though communication skills are more than language, as many mute children show, using only the power of pointing to get everything they need, language is the essential foundation of human communication. A delay or disturbance of language development can be the first sign of possible autism, since language has a different function for autistic people than NT people. And because of the lack of imitation of the other person, it also has to be learned differently.

For NT people, language is less about transmitting information, but about 60 percent of "social grooming". Through language, the imitation of speech melody and dialects ..., unconsciously the group affiliation is communicated.

For autistics, however, language is above all the exchange of factual information. Autistic children like to tell about their areas of interest, ask questions of knowledge, often to the limits of parents and educators. Autistic children are also interested in people, but more in people who can and want to explain the world to them.

Therefore, in the promotion of language of autistic children, the interests of the child should be chosen as exercise objects.

3   Promotion of social (!) interaction

Due to the lack of unconscious group communication and the resulting problems, autistic children often withdraw from social interaction. Or they are marginalized, for example, because of their strong exploration behavior or the mistaken belief that autistics can not and do not want to be part of social interaction.

But social interaction can be learned by participating in groups, by participating in social interaction.

For all children, particular attention must be paid to anxiety and stress, as fear and stress stand in the way of social interaction. For "flight" children, who retreat into their own world, into their own games and stereotypes, careful approach to the group interaction is necessary.

For the "fighting" children, their exploration of the environment can be used to build social interaction by allowing exploration, accompanying children and explaining "the world" to them.

4 Sensitivity to bullying / violence

In addition to the risk of overstrain due to insufficiently developed interaction skills, autistic people also have a far greater than average risk of becoming victims of bullying, violence and exploitation. Socio-psychologically, this is explained by the fact that people who are not part of the self-group are perceived as foreign and / or hostile. Due to the lack of unconscious group communication, especially without imitation of dialects, fashions, etc., autistic people are hardly or not at all perceived as members of the self-group. As a result, they are perceived as "strangers" and treated as such.

VII.   IS A CHILD AUTISTIC?

The following points are intended to provide guidance in answering the question of whether a child is autistic. And this at a time when there is no or so little disruption of development that it is insufficient for a diagnosis (a profound developmental disorder).

- In comparison to other children little to no facial expressions

Autistic people show little to no facial expressions. This is one of the main criteria for identifying autistic children and adolescents.

However, some adult autistic individuals have learned to express facial expressions.

- No imitation

Autists do not imitate the behavior of other people.

- No fear

Even fear is learned socially. Without appropriate social interaction, there is no development of culture-specific anxiety.

On the other hand, autistic people have a high risk of developing an anxiety disorder.

- No "pretend play", tractors are lined up

Autistic children do not show a "pretend play". Toy tractors are small images of the great reality. These are mainly sorted.

- Interest in things / nature. Better a non-fiction book than a storybook.

- Strong exploration or withdrawal

- Sensory

The sensory perception of autistic children is often divided into two parts. For one thing exists
        - hardly pain perception and interoception.
On the other hand, with the sensory stimuli one
        - Hypersensitivity

- motor skills

Autistic children can be recognized by the unusual
movement patterns. Frequently, this also sports deficits
appear. The children have often
- "wooden" movements.
On the other hand, but also found
- "Klettermax", that means astonishing skill in
climbing, for example
- good eye-hand coordination
In principle, have autists
- high activity / arousal levels.
These may be manifested by a spasticity-like posture of
the hands and arms, as well as teeth grinding, muscle
tension ...

- language

Without the imitation of the speech melody, autistic
language is often monotone. Due to the restriction on the
subject content, it often comes to the "little professor"
communication.

VIII.   EPILOGUE

Autism is not a disease!

Autism is another form of being.

This is accompanied in our cultural environment by a particularly high risk of disrupting social interaction through withdrawal or exclusion.

And as a result, it can then lead to a disruption of development.

If this is heeded and an autistic child recognized as such in time, then it can develop as normal with appropriate understanding, appropriate support and sensitivity to the stress balance!

IX. FURTHER READING

Schmidt, Bernhard J. (2015/1): Autistic and Society. An angry Change of Perspective. Vol. I: Understanding Autism. Norderstedt: Books on Demand.

Schmidt, Bernhard J. (2015/2): Autistic and Society. An angry Change of Perspective. Vol. II: Support for Autistic? Norderstedt: Books on Demand.

Schmidt, Bernhard J. (2016/1): Plaintext compact. The Asperger Syndrome – Between Bullying and Inclusion. Norderstedt: Books on Demand.

Schmidt, Bernhard J. (2016/2):
Autismus. Wenn Händewaschen hilft.
1. Auflage. Norderstedt: Books on Demand

Schmidt, Bernhard J. (2019/1): Autism and the Refrigerator Mother Myth. A Rehabilitation of Bruno Bettelheim. Norderstedt: Books on Demand.

Schmidt, Bernhard J. (2019/2): Plaintext compact. The Asperger Syndrome – for Parents. Norderstedt: Books on Demand.

Schmidt, Bernhard J. (2019/3): Plaintext compact. The Asperger Syndrome – for Teachers. Norderstedt: Books on Demand.

Schmidt, Bernhard J. (2019/4): Plaintext compact. The Asperger Syndrome – for School Assistants. Norderstedt: Books on Demand.

Schmidt, Bernhard J. (2019/5): Autism – Flight or Fight. New Perspectives on Challenging Behaviors. Norderstedt: Books on Demand.

Schmidt, Bernhard J.; Döhler, Christiane and Deniz (2018): Autism – Sexuality – Relationships. Norderstedt: Books on Demand.

Schmidt, Bernhard J.; Ganz, Andreas (2016): Plaintext compact: The Asperger Syndrome - not only for Psychotherapists. Norderstedt: Books on Demand.

Schmidt, Bernhard J.; Ganz, Andreas (2019/6): Plaintext compact. The Asperger Syndrome – for Physicians. Norderstedt: Books on Demand.